A DAY AT THE BEACH

BY
JAMIE STONEBRIDGE

ALSO BY JAMIE STONEBRIDGE

Trip To The Lake
A Day At The Park
A Visit To The Farm
A Day At The Beach

And more...

amazon.com/author/jamiestonebridge

THANK YOU

It is people like you that keep reading alive.
We can all live through books. Reading alone
or with others is a wonderful thing.

I hope this book brings you joy and
happiness.

You can help other readers discover this book
by leaving a review on Amazon.

Special thanks to Misty Gardener. Without
her, none of this would be possible.

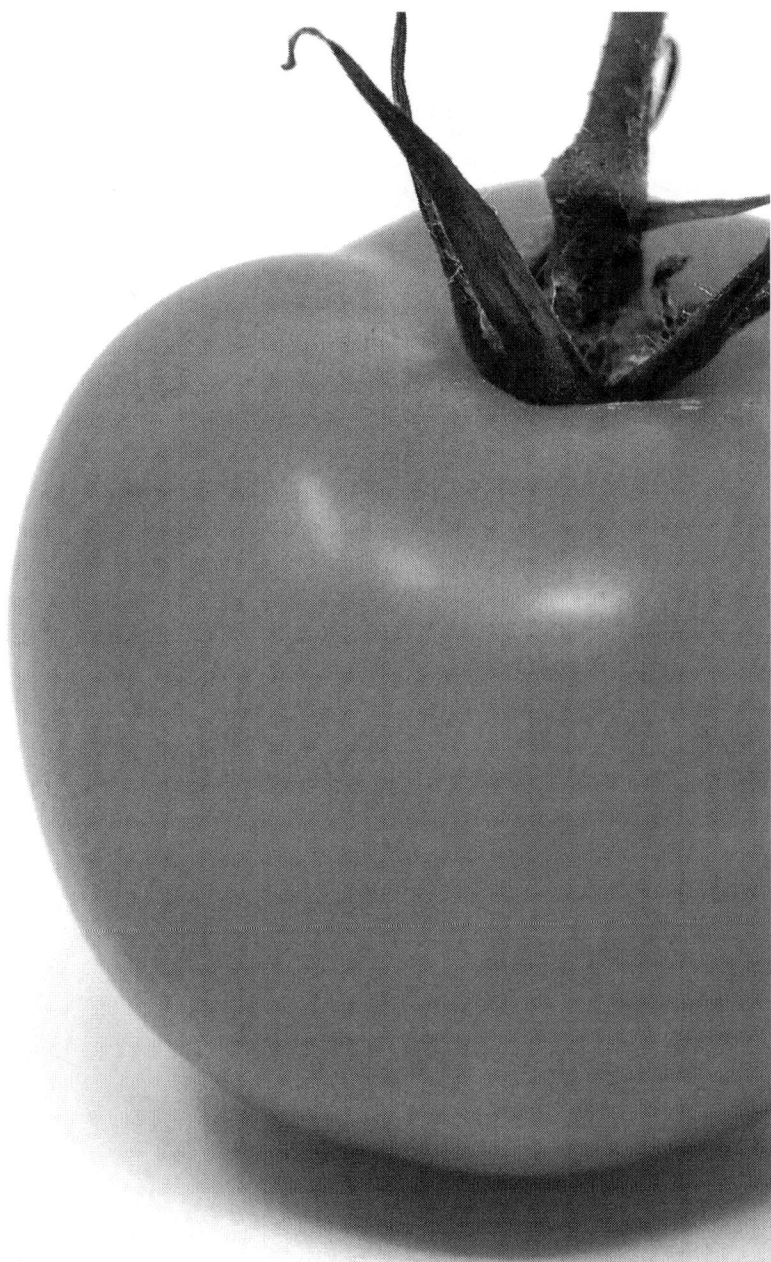

CHAPTER 1
A Good Idea

THE TABLE IS piled high with red ripe strawberries, sweet slices of watermelon, and plump, juicy blueberries. I pull out my chair and sit down to enjoy my lunch. David places a delicate china plate in front of me. The plate holds a tall sandwich full of ham, Swiss cheese, lettuce, and tomato. The tomato was grown in our own backyard and looks smooth and perfect.

"Thank you," I say to David. "This looks delicious."

I pick up the pickle spear that lies beside my giant sandwich and bite into it. The salty tang of vinegar and seasoning hits my mouth and makes my throat tingle as I swallow.

David joins me at the table, his own plate weighed down with a sandwich that looks like mine. We are sitting together on the sun porch, enjoying the warm summer sunlight while we eat our lunch.

"How does it taste?" David asks.

I have just taken a big bite of my sandwich. Tangy tomato juice runs down my chin and drips onto the yellow tablecloth. Crumbs from the toasted bread also fall to dot the table. I close my eyes and savor the taste.

"It is yummy. I am so glad you suggested that we plant tomatoes this year. It really makes this sandwich delicious," I say to David once my mouth is empty.

Outside, a gentle summer breeze makes the leaves on our oak tree shimmer. I watch the pattern of sunlight on the sidewalk shift as the leaves bend and sway. David stands up and opens the door. As soon as he does, the breeze blows past me, ruffling my hair and sweeping a napkin to the floor.

"It is such a beautiful day today. I think we should go somewhere," I say to David as I bend to pick up the fallen napkin.

He nods his head and looks out the window for a moment. "How about the beach?" he asks.

My heart leaps. The beach is one of my favorite places to spend time. I am always ready for a trip to the beach. David and I are lucky; we only live about an hour from a lovely little beach.

"Yes!" I say. "As soon as we finish eating, let's pack our bags and go. What a great idea, David."

I finish the food left on my plate and plan in my mind what I should bring on this trip. I will certainly wear my blue bathing suit. I will also need to remember to bring a towel, some sunscreen, and a book to read. I begin to get very excited. This will be my first beach trip of the summer. It has been far too long since I've seen the ocean and felt the sand crunch between my toes.

David clears the table and washes our two plates while I head off into the bedroom to pack my things. I take my large canvas bag from the high shelf in the closet. The bag's handles are made of rope and it has a picture of an anchor on the side. It is a perfect bag for a day at the beach.

I put a spray bottle of sunscreen in the side pocket and roll up a bright pink towel. The towel is a gift from an old friend. My birthday was last month, and she knows how much I enjoy the beach, so a huge towel was really a thoughtful gift for me. There is just enough room left in the bag for my paperback book, a pair of sunglasses, and my cell phone.

I slip my bathing suit on and pull an old t-shirt over my head as a cover-up.

"David? Are you ready?" I yell down the hall, as excited as a kid on the first day of summer vacation. He pokes his head around the corner and smiles at me.

"Yep. All ready." He slings his own tote bag over his shoulder and walks down the hall to meet me.

"Let's go, dear," he says and links his arm through mine.

"I think we'll take the convertible today."

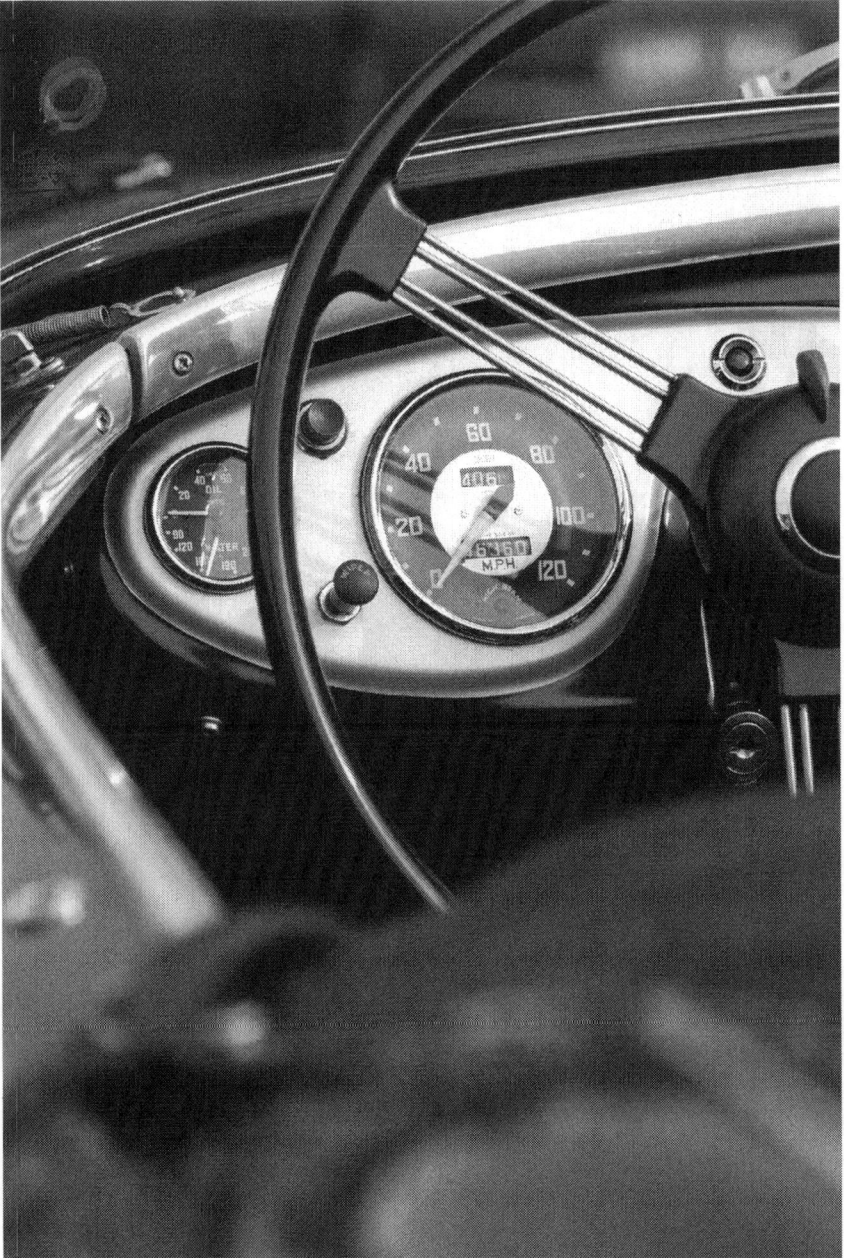

CHAPTER 2
Slow Ride

I AM SO EXCITED at the idea of riding in David's convertible. It is a beautiful car. It is shiny black on the outside with smooth gray leather seats inside. He washes and waxes it every week, so the car is always in good condition.

I stand on the porch and watch as David backs the car out of the garage slowly. I place my hand above my eyes to block out the blinding sun so that I can see better. David parks in the driveway and I see the trunk pop open.

"Are you packed and ready?" he calls to me as he slides out of the car. I look down at myself. Blue bathing suit - check. Flip-flops - check. I look in my beach bag one last time to make sure I haven't forgotten anything.

"I think I'm all ready," I answer. I walk down the porch steps with my bag over one shoulder. David is back in the garage lifting beach chairs off of hooks on the wall. The chairs are the kind that are low to the ground. I like to sit in them at the ocean's edge and let the water wash over my feet.

David carries one chair in each hand and puts them in the car's trunk. I lift my bag up and set it on top of the chairs. I feel as happy as a child on vacation.

"Where is your bag, David?" I ask.

"Just inside the house. Let me grab it and lock the door then we can get going."

He opens the passenger door for me and I ease myself down into the comfortable seat. David leans across me and pushes a button on the dash. He grins at me and hurries off to get his things from inside the house. I hear an electric hum and the roof of the car begins to slide back.

Golden sunlight splashes onto my lap and warms my face as the gap in the car's top widens. Once the roof is open all the way the car becomes quiet. I lay my head back against the seat and close my eyes. I slide my sunglasses on and wait for David to return.

Only a moment later, I hear the trunk click shut and then David is beside me turning the key and cranking the car.

"Here we come, beach," he says.

David honks the horn and waves as we pass our neighbor's house. Our neighbor is outside watering his grass. I lift my hand to wave also as we roll slowly down the quiet street. Once we're out of the neighborhood, David reaches down and turns on the radio. Upbeat music fills my ears and I bob my head and shoulders along with the beat.

Soon we're on the highway driving fast, the wind blowing my short hair back off my face. We have turned the music up louder to hear it over the rush of the wind and I am still dancing in my seat. In no time, I smell a hint of salt in the air and, as David rounds a curve, the long, winding coastline comes into view.

On this coast, there are very few hotels and only a few houses, so the view is clear. The road we're on runs high above the beach so I feel as if I can see for miles. I look down at the crystal blue water and can't wait to jump in. Soft white waves gently flow over the sand as I watch. The ocean is calm today. It is perfect for swimming.

David slows the car and turns on the turn signal. He pulls into a sandy little parking lot between two houses. The warm ocean breeze blows sand back and forth across the pavement.

"I'd better put the top up quickly before the whole car is full of sand," David says and pushes the button. I wait until it is closed to open the door and step out. Tiny grains of sand sting my ankles and feet as I walk around to the back of the car. I slip my flip-flops off my feet and slide them down into my beach bag. David kicks off his own shoes and wiggles his toes down into a pile of sand.

Barefoot is the only way to walk onto a beach.

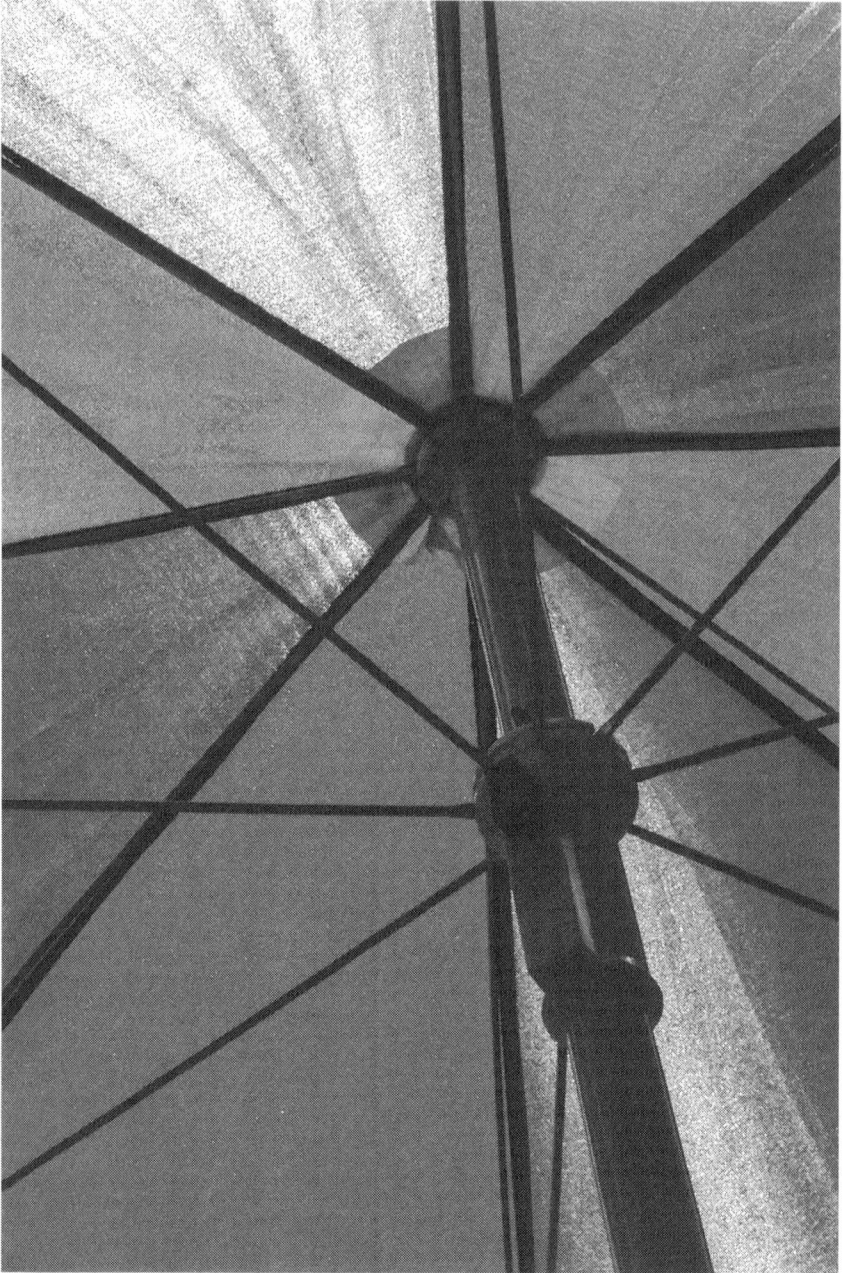

CHAPTER 3
Sand Between Our Toes

DAVID LIFTS OUR chairs out of the car and underneath I notice for the first time that he's also packed a colorful beach umbrella. He picks this up as well and begins to make his clumsy way down to the beach.

"Here, let me carry something," I say and hold out my empty hand. He gratefully passes one of the chairs to me and we continue our search for an empty spot where we can settle our things.

It is Saturday and the beach is pretty crowded. Everywhere there are pockets of people enjoying the beautiful sunny day. I let my eyes roam over the scene and I see a perfect little spot for two people. I tell David to follow me and I lead us almost to the water's edge.

A seagull dips down from the sky and lands on the sand near my feet. He bends his head to snap up someone's discarded potato chip. The bird squawks and waddles closer to me.

"Shoo!" I say. "We don't have any potato chips to share. You're out of luck." I wave my hand at the bird to scare him away but he just stands and stares at me. I shrug and turn my attention to setting up my chair.

I sit down to test it out and giggle as the cold foamy water bubbles over my bare toes. The water is colder than I expected but it is a nice contrast to the hot sun. David sits down beside me with a sigh and for a moment we are just quiet.

"Let's enjoy the sun a bit before we set up the umbrella, ok?" I ask. David nods. I wiggle my feet side to side until they are completely buried under the sand. With each coming wave, the pile of sand is washed away. I enjoy the sensation.

In the distance, just beyond the reach of the waves, a large blue fishing boat bobs on the ocean. I watch as a tall man stands on the front of the boat, gathering something in his arms. In one quick motion, he sends a giant fishing net sailing out into the water. It sinks out of sight for a moment. Another man joins the tall man at the front of the boat and together they begin to drag the net back out of the water.

Even though the men are far away I can see the muscles in their arms standing out as they lift the heavy net from the sea. It is now full of wiggling silver-scaled fish. As the fish flop against each other in the net, their scales blink in the bright sunlight and remind me of a disco ball. Finally, the men get the net all the way in the boat and I can no longer see the fish. There is a distant hum as the boat's motor starts back up and one man steers it further away from shore.

By this time the sun is beginning to sink into my skin. I feel the familiar burn of its rays. I reach into my bag and take out a little bottle of sunscreen. As I spray it on my arms and legs, its coconut smell reminds me of childhood vacations long past and fun times with my friends when we were younger.

"Isn't this nice?" I ask David. He mumbles a response, seeming to be half asleep already.

"Here, you better put some of this on if you're going to nap out here," I say and pass the bottle of sunscreen over to him.

"Thanks," he says, taking the bottle. I shield my eyes and make sure to keep my mouth closed as he sprays his arms. It may smell delicious, but it definitely doesn't taste good!

A gust of wind brings a bright red bucket tumbling up to my feet. I quickly reach down to grab it and look around for its owner. A little boy, about six years old, runs up to me. He is out of breath and a lady who must be his mother is trailing along behind him.

"Is this yours?" I ask him, holding out the bucket.

He nods his little blond head and takes the bucket from me.

"I'm building the biggest sandcastle on the whole beach," he says and makes a grand movement with his arms.

"Well, I would love to see it when you're done."

"Ok, me and my mom are right back here," he says, pointing to a spot not far behind us.

"Ok, you come let me know when you're finished and I'll come see it."

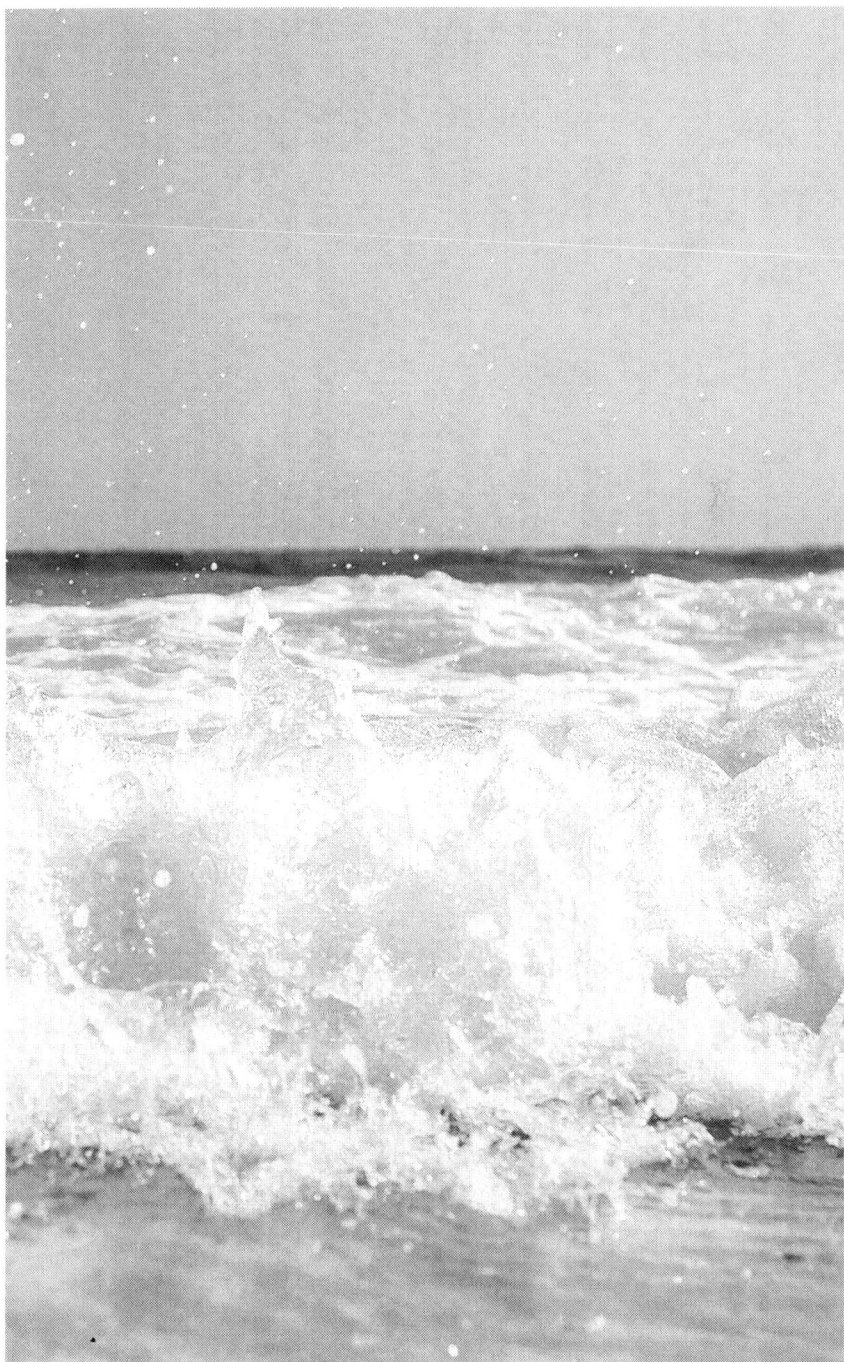

CHAPTER 4
Into the Surf

THE BOY SKIPS off, swinging his bucket and kicking up little sprays of sand behind his feet. By this time, I am quite hot and ready to take a swim.

I stand up from my chair and with only a few steps I am knee-deep in the salty water. I try to keep my balance as wave after wave sucks the sand from under my feet. David laughs as I wobble and throw my arms out to the side for balance.

I walk on into the ocean and am now waist deep. I pick up my feet and let the water hold me.

There are people in the water next to me and I hear small pieces of conversation as I bob up and down. A family with a baby float beside me. The baby sits in a little boat shaped like a frog. She pats the frog's green head and happily splashes her tiny feet in the water. I love her laugh. I smile at her mother and father and swim deeper into the sea.

When the water reaches my chest, I stop. This time, I pick my feet all the way up to the water's surface and let myself float on my back. I feel like a kid again.

I let my arms fall out to the side of my body

and just give myself to the ocean. It is so peaceful. My ears are under the water so all is quiet. Gently, my body dips up and down on the calm ocean.

A piece of slimy green seaweed has wrapped around my arm. I watch it wave in the water for a second before pulling it off.

After a moment, I stand back up and wave to David so he will join me. He waves back and I see him stand from his chair. He holds up one finger to tell me to wait and he walks to a stand at the back of the beach. In this area, there are toys, chairs, food, drinks, and other things for sale.

I cannot see what David is doing but it becomes clear when he walks into the water to meet me. He has a bright green float tucked under each arm. Each one is long enough to lie on and I am happy he has brought them into the water.

My legs are getting tired and I am thankful for a float to sit on in the water.

"It will be easier to get on this in the shallow water," David says. We walk toward the beach and I find he is right. I swing my leg over the float and plop down. Somehow, I manage to not fall off. I use my legs to push myself back out into the deeper water. Once I can no longer touch the bottom, I lie back and get comfortable on the float.

David suggests we hold hands so we don't float apart. I agree that this is a good idea. As I lie on the float and look up at the sky I see two large birds fly over our heads. I think I remember what they're called. Pelicans. The birds have very large pouches below their beaks. As I watch, one of them swoops down into the water to catch a fish.

The water that drips from the bird's beak glitters in the sun and looks beautiful. I hope he caught himself a nice lunch, I think. Thinking of the bird eating makes my stomach growl.

"Are you getting hungry?" I ask David.

"Yes, a little," he says. "I packed some crackers and fruit in my bag. When we get ready to get out we can have a little snack. Sound good?"

"Yep. That's works for me," I reply.

I'm not quite hungry enough to go back to the beach just yet. I am perfectly relaxed bobbing in the gentle waves.

As I look towards the beach, I notice the little blond boy building his sandcastle. He is happily sitting, covered in sand, in the middle of dozens of small mounds. Even from the water, I can see bright flags fluttering on top of them. His mother is sitting nearby reading a book.

I enjoy watching them for a minute and remember making my own sandcastles.

I also think back on long ago vacations where my friends and I would get sunburns from staying in the water so long. We would talk about everything you could imagine and would never want to come in.

Being at the beach always makes me wish I lived at the beach. As we float, I daydream about just that. I picture a cute little beach cottage with a front porch swing facing the water. I would love to spend my evenings sitting on that porch, watching the sunset over the water.

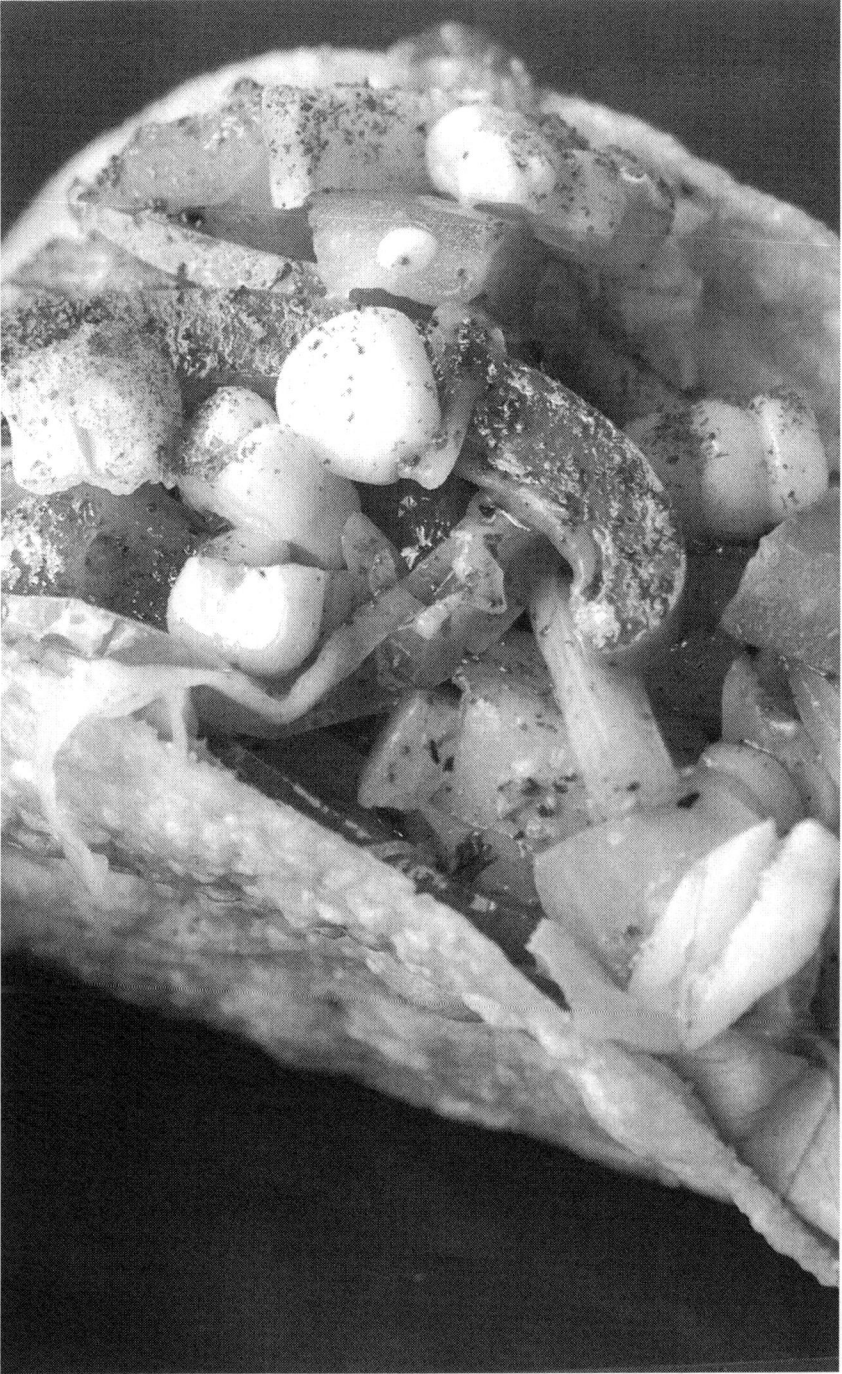

CHAPTER 5
Time to Eat

SOON I BEGIN to notice a new smell in the salty air. I raise my head and scan the beach to see where it is coming from. It doesn't take long to find the source of the delicious smell. A brightly colored truck sits parked at the back of the beach. A picture of a cartoon taco decorates the side of the truck. There is also a window that slides open. I can see people moving around and cooking inside.

Yellow, green, and blue flags wave in the wind

on top of the truck. I see a line beginning to form in front of the open window.

"Ok, I'm definitely hungry now," I say. "I think we should swim back to the beach and get some tacos."

"Tacos?" David mumbles and I can see he was almost asleep on his float. He lifts his head now too and looks at where I'm pointing. I can see by the look on his face that the delicious smell has reached him also.

The smell is full of rich spices and the warm scent of meat cooking on a buttered grill. I think I can smell peppers and onions as well. I can see steam rising from a vent in the top of the truck.

David breathes in deeply and makes a silly

face. He licks his lips and rubs his hand over his stomach and nods.

"My belly is telling me that tacos sound like a great idea," he says, "forget the boring crackers and fruit. Let's get some real food!"

We both swing our legs over the sides of our floats and begin half-walking, half-swimming back to the shore. We let the strong waves push against our backs and use that force to speed up our trip back to the sand.

My own stomach begins to rumble as we get closer. Walking gets harder as the water gets more shallow so David and I lean on one another to keep from falling down. I am sure we look pretty funny as we stumble over the uneven sand.

I lift my legs high to try to step over the waves and not get pulled back into the deeper water. In this clumsy way, we finally make it out of the water. We stack our floats beside our chairs and dry ourselves off a little. I roll my towel back up and put it back in my bag so it doesn't get covered in sand. David pulls his wallet out of his bag.

"I'm starving all of a sudden," he says as we make our way to the end of the line at the taco truck.

There are only four people in line ahead of us, so our wait is not very long. I read the menu as we stand and decide I will order a chicken and cheese taco with sour cream, refried beans and avocado on top. My mouth waters just thinking about it.

When it is our turn, I let David place our order. The lady at the window asks if we want anything to drink. An ice-cold Coca-Cola sounds perfect to me, so I tell her so.

On the right side of the truck, there are four picnic tables. One is empty, so we get our food and go sit. We can watch our belongings from here and have a more comfortable place to eat. Next to us, a family of five laughs and talks loudly. They seem to be having such a good time I can't help but smile at them.

A little boy smiles back at me and waves his chubby hand. I wave at him and continue eating my taco.

It is not long before all our food is gone and our bellies are stuffed. We clean up our trash and throw it in the garbage can.

It has been such a nice afternoon so far. David and I walk back to our chairs and settle in to soak up some more sun. The food and sun together have made me sleepy. I let my mind rest as I watch two kites fly in the breeze. One is shaped like a dragon. Its tail is made of rainbow-colored streamers that trail behind it in the strong wind.

I trace the line down from the sky to a girl who looks about fourteen years old. She holds tightly to the kite handle and runs along the beach, splashing in the edge of the water and kicking up sand behind her bare feet. My eyes begin to close as she gets further away and for a while, I just doze.

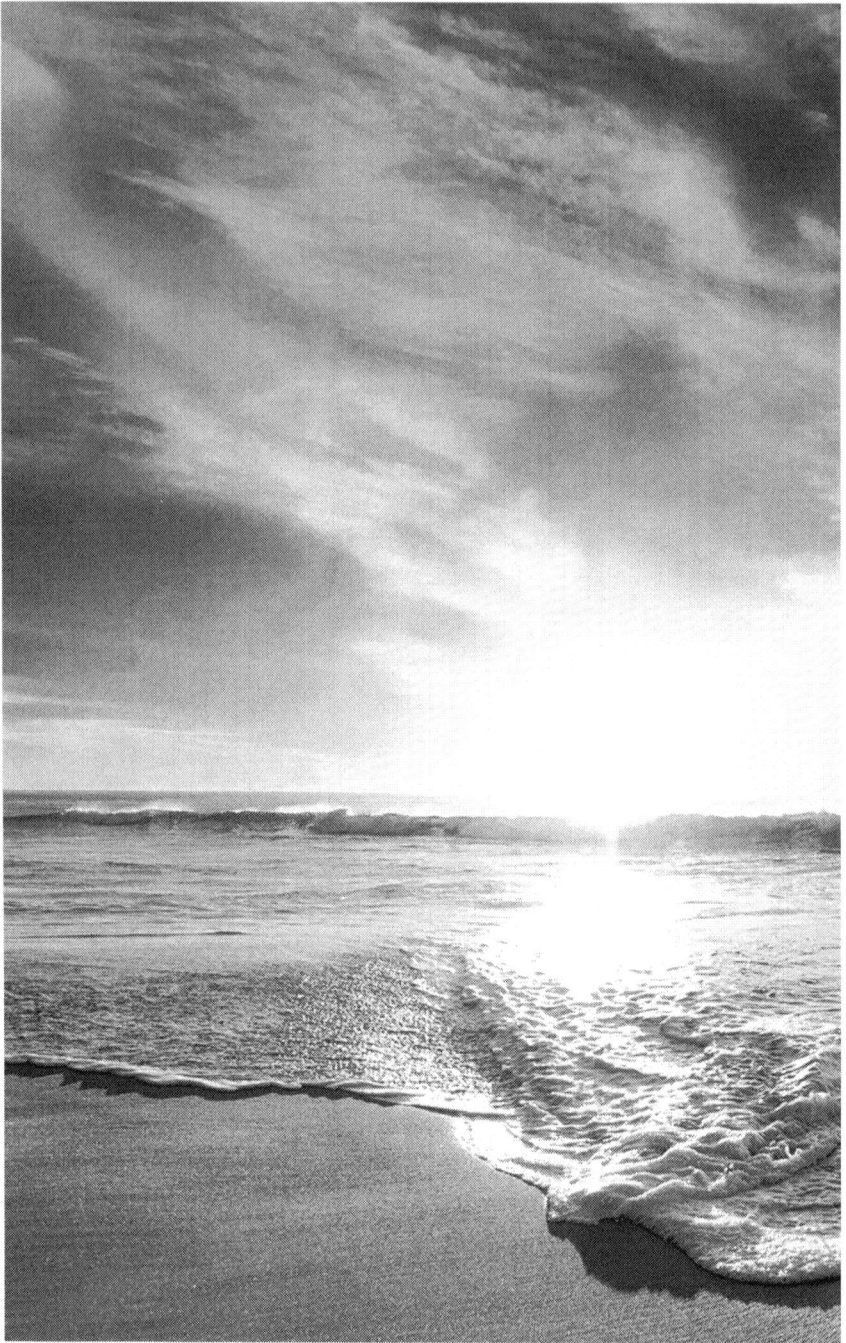

CHAPTER 6
Sunset

I HAVE ENJOYED so many wonderful memories at the beach today. Happy family memories of vacations as a child, good times with friends, and the pleasure of making new memories now.

It doesn't seem possible that our afternoon is coming to an end, but as I sit in my chair and watch the ocean I see the sun sinking closer and closer to the water.

The setting sun has turned the clouds a million beautiful colors. Pink and purple fluff floating gently across a darkening sky. I slide my sunglasses up on my head so that I can take in this amazing sight more clearly. The sun is close enough to the water now that it appears to be melting into the sea. It spreads its orange fire along the far edge of the water.

"Look," David whispers to me.

I look out into the ocean and can see a pod of dolphins playing. I see their smooth bodies leap out of the water, one after another. It looks as if there are about five of them. They swim so fast they quickly move out of sight, but it is such a joy to see them splashing around.

"Oh, how amazing," I say. "I haven't seen

dolphins here since I was a kid."

David smiles at me. "Have you enjoyed yourself today?" he asks.

"Very much," I answer.

"Me too. I think it is about time to pack up and head home though, don't you?"

"Yes. I suppose we should. It will be dark soon."

I stand up and begin to gather my belongings. David does the same. We take extra care to not leave anything behind.

I take one last long look at the sky and the water and the beach. I breathe in deeply one more time and feel so content with myself.

On our way out, we pass a group of young people gathered around a small bonfire. They laugh and talk in loud voices. I see the girls toss their long hair in the firelight and see the boys doing stunts and flips on the sand to impress those girls. I think back to being that young.

There is a shower head attached to a post near the parking area. David and I stop to rinse our feet and legs before we get in his car. The water is colder than the ocean and gives me goosebumps. I pat my feet dry with my pink towel and slide my flip-flops back on my feet.

Once we have loaded the trunk we climb in and begin the drive back home. I watch out the window as the sky continues to fade from blue to gray to black.

"Thanks for taking me to the beach today," I say to David. He nods and pats my knee.

"It was a lot of fun," he says.

We pull into the driveway and unload our things. David hangs the chairs back on their hooks and I throw our towels and bathing suits in the washing machine. Once those chores are completed, I walk upstairs to take a nice warm shower.

There is no other feeling that compares to the feel of your skin after a nice day at the beach. The sand has smoothed the rough parts and the sun has given me a little glow. I study myself in the mirror before stepping into the shower and am filled with happiness again.

The shower is so warm on my sunbaked skin that I just stand there under the spray and let the sand and sweat slide off my body.

I look forward to sliding between my crisp, clean sheets tonight. The sun has a way of zapping your energy and making you tired in a very special way.

My day at the beach has been very special. Time spent with those you love is always a good thing. I know I will fall into a deep, contented sleep tonight replaying the day in my head.

Made in the USA
San Bernardino, CA
17 November 2019